Fitness with the Buddha

Spiritual Practices for Physical Well-Being

Table of Contents

Chapter 1. Introduction

Venture on a unique journey of holistic well-being with our special report on "Fitness with the Buddha: Spiritual Practices for Physical Well-Being". This inviting blend of spirituality and physical fitness will comfortably guide you through ancient wisdom and modern fitness advice, which together, promises a path towards not just physical health, but also inner tranquility. Be ready to engage your body, mind, and soul in a harmonious dance of wellness, where robust workouts meet meditative practices, infusing your fitness regimen with a sublime depth. Experience health not as a tedious routine, but as joyous living. Order this report today, and embark upon a path leading not just to a healthier body, but also a more peaceful and focused mind!

Chapter 2. Embracing the Path of Buddha: An Introduction

Unraveling the teachings of the Enlightened One, one of the world's earliest proponents of mental and physical health, forms an essential aspect of our quest for holistic well-being. Consequently, as we embrace the path of Buddha, we shall translate and integrate the healer's 2,500-year-old wisdom into a fitness regimen fit for the 21st Century, focused on nourishing not just the body, but the mind and soul as well.

2.1. The Buddha's Philosophy

Akin to the principles underpinning physical health, Buddha's philosophy, hinging on meanings beyond the mere physical existence, originates from understanding the nature of suffering. Buddha, also known as Siddhartha Gautama, embarked on a spiritual journey, meditating under the Bodhi tree until he attained complete enlightenment. This process of self-discovery led him to identify the Four Noble Truths, explaining the existence of suffering, its origin, cessation, and the path leading to cessation.

Embedded within this profound understanding lies the essence of maintaining physical well-being. The Buddha's teachings reinforce the necessity of a disciplined regimen for maintaining physical health, one of the significant pillars of his 'Middle Path.' The Buddha appreciated the gravity of physical fitness as profoundly as his emphasis on spiritual well-being.

2.2. Eudaimonia and Physical Fitness: The Buddhist Perspective

The Buddha reasoned that a sound body houses a sound mind, underscoring the criticality of physical health. Yet, he cautioned against extreme measures, whether in the form of self-indulgence or self-mortification. This 'Middle Path' echoes the Greek concept of 'Eudaimonia,' advocating for individual well-being and happiness derived from virtuous acts, including exercise and nurturing the physical form. This notion of balance—even while fostering physical well-being—lies at the heart of the Buddha's teaching.

2.3. The Middle Path to Fitness

The Buddha's Middle Path offers an antidote to the hyperactive grind of modern life, marked by excesses of hedonism or asceticism. Herein lies the balance, striving neither for over-indulgence nor total denial but a judicious combination of diet, physical activity, and mental exercises. This 'Middle Path' carries immense relevance to curating a balanced fitness regimen that harmonizes the requirements of the body with those of the mind and soul.

2.4. The Eightfold Path: Exploring the Spiritual Aspects

Notably, Buddha's Eightfold Path concentrates primarily on ethical behavior, wisdom, and mental discipline, offering directives for right view, right resolve, right speech, right conduct, right livelihood, right effort, right mindfulness, and right meditation. Astonishingly, these truths can act as guiding principles for our fitness journey, urging us towards ethical eating habits, righteous methods of maintaining fitness, and an overall balance.

Guiding this exploration, we unmask the mystery of the Four Noble Truths and Eightfold Path through the lens of physical well-being, bridging spirituality, mindfulness and fitness. This convergence promises an entrancing amalgamation of insights drawn from the ancient wisdom, coupled with the science of maintaining physical health, broadly defining our scope to cultivate a mindful fitness regimen.

2.5. Infusing Wisdom into our Fitness Journey

Given the depth and breadth of the Buddha's teaching, one might ask - how could these bedrocks of Buddhism influence our fitness journey? The answer lies in understanding the interplay of various principles of Buddhist teachings and mindfulness, illustrating their relevance in the pursuit of physical fitness. From adapting a conscious diet (Right Livelihood) to employing a disciplined approach to physical activity (Right Effort), the Buddhist teachings guide us towards good health with a rounded sense of well-being.

Expanding from this base understanding, we further delve into specific aspects of the fitness regimen, shedding light on a unique meditative workout session, relaxing yoga postures inspired by Buddhism, and a specially curated Buddhist diet, all motivated by the principles of the Middle Path.

Through this chapter, we hope to enlighten readers on the interconnectedness of the physical and spiritual realms inspired by Buddha's wisdom. By integrating the Buddha's teachings into the core of our fitness routine, we not only sculpt a healthier body but also meld a more mindful way of life, balanced and nourished in every dimension.

Chapter 3. Spirituality and Physical Fitness: The Connection

The interconnectedness of mind, body, and spirit is a widely accepted concept in holistic wellness. This harmony between different aspects of your being is intrinsic to understanding the symbiosis between physical fitness and spirituality. In the next few pages, we delve deeper into this fascinating connection, introducing a fresh perspective on physical well-being that extends beyond appearances and calisthenics.

3.1. The Spectrum of Well-being: More than Physical Fitness

When we talk about fitness, we often limit ourselves to the realm of physical prowess – strength, flexibility, and endurance. And in doing that, we overlook the fundamental fact that us human beings are not solely physical entities. We consist of emotional, mental, and spiritual dimensions that are as critical to our overall health as our physical state. When we integrate these dimensions into our fitness goals, we pursue well-being in its truest, holistic sense. A truly fit person is not just physically adept, but also emotionally balanced, mentally strong, and spiritually awakened.

Before we delve into the correlation between physical fitness and spirituality, it is essential to take a moment and contemplate what 'spirituality' means. Spirituality is the consciousness of a sacred, transcendent dimension beyond our mundane realities – a sense of connection to something larger than oneself. It often involves personal growth, self-realization, and the pursuit of higher states of consciousness.

3.2. Symbiosis of the Physical and the Spiritual

The human body is the vessel that houses our spirit, making it an inseparable part of our spiritual journey. Just like a well-functioning car makes a road trip more enjoyable, a healthy, robust physique can enhance our spiritual journey.

Such a symbiotic relationship between physical health and spirituality isn't abstract or conjectural, but backed by science. Various scientific studies have revealed that regular physical activity can lower stress, anxiety, and depression–all of which clutter our spiritual path.

Likewise, spirituality can have profound effects on physical health. Practices like meditation, mindfulness, and yoga designed to cultivate spirituality have been shown to control blood pressure, boost the immune system, and improve cardiovascular health, thus contributing to physical health.

3.3. Pathways of Connection

While the body-spirit connection may seem foreign and elusive, several religious, philosophical, and wellness traditions have long acknowledged this link. These traditions have developed methodologies that marry physical activity with spiritual discipline.

One such path is Yoga. Originating from ancient India, Yoga, meaning 'union,' is a practice designed to unify the mind, body, and spirit. By performing various postures (asanas), controlling breath (pranayama), and meditating (dhyana), a practitioner can attain physical fitness, mental clarity, and spiritual awakening.

Buddhism, particularly Zen, is another tradition that underscores the body-spirit connection. Zazen, or seated meditation, is a widely practiced Zen ritual that advocates the importance of posture in achieving enlightenment.

Prostrations, a common practice across various religions, is yet another example of spiritual traditions utilizing physical activity to propel spiritual growth.

3.4. The Intersection of Physical Exercise and Meditation

Physical exercise and meditation, though seemingly disparate, share common ground and can complement one another. By incorporating mindfulness, a form of meditation, into your physical workouts, you can deepen your physical activities' effects, transforming them into a spiritual routine.

When we exercise mindlessly, we often dissociate our mind from our body, viewing pain or discomfort as an adversary. However, when we bring mindfulness into exercise, we learn to notice and accept feelings of exertion, discomfort, or even pain, instead of resisting them. This practice of mindfulness can transform physical exercises into a meditative process, making us more in tune with our bodies and the present moment.

3.5. Enhancing Physical Fitness with Spiritual Practices

Reaping the benefits of this holistic approach to fitness involves incorporating spiritual practices into your existing workout routine.

Practices such as yoga, Tai Chi, and Qigong are excellent ways to balance physical vitality with spiritual enlightenment. These practices focus on mindful movements, deep breathing, and meditation, promoting a sense of peace, enhancing focus, and leading to a holistic form of fitness.

Equally beneficial is the practice of outdoor workouts in nature's lap. The serene surroundings can help deepen your mindfulness practice and nourish your spirituality by fostering a sense of interconnectedness with the Universe.

Chapter 4. Embracing the Journey

Remember, the aim is not just a fit body but a harmoniously functioning human being, vibrant in every sense. When physical fitness routines are combined with spiritual practices, they can form a formidable alliance against physical ailments and existential dilemmas.

Embrace this journey of holistic fitness embracing both the physical and spiritual disciplines. As your body becomes stronger, leaner, and more efficient, you'll find your mind becoming more peaceful, your heart becoming more open, and your spirit soaring high.

By nurturing your physical self and spiritual self simultaneously, you can reach unprecedented levels of well-being. So, step onto this path of integrated wellness today, and uncover the 'fit and tranquil' YOU waiting to unfold!

Chapter 5. Body as the Temple: Transformative Workouts

As we embark on this transformative journey, it is vital to comprehend the perspective that our bodies are temples. They are the magnificent vessels that carry our souls, minds, and the precious gift of life itself. Attuning ourselves to this wisdom helps engender a profound respect and care for our bodies.

5.1. Understanding Your Temple

In order to refine and nurture our temples, the first critical step is understanding. A foundation should be built upon solid knowledge of the structure, dynamics, and needs of the physical body.

The human body is a complex system consisting of several organ systems such as the skeletal, muscular, cardiovascular, respiratory, digestive, and nervous systems. Each of these function in harmony to facilitate our daily actions, reactions, and existence. Understanding the basic functionality of these systems is vital as it enables us to foster an awareness of our body's boundaries, strengths, and potential areas of improvement. It is valuable to consult a healthcare provider or fitness professional to ascertain your body's current condition and to identify any potential limitations or areas that require special caution.

5.2. Respect and Nurture Your Body

Viewing the body as a sacred temple calls for mindful nurturing. We are not just talking about a basic level of care that wards off ailments. Instead, our objective is to help your body thrive, rather than simply survive.

Eating nutritious, well-balanced meals, staying hydrated, and getting enough rest are immediate steps one can take. It is also recommended to keep stimulants & toxins at bay as much as possible. Electing to consume organic foods whenever possible, reducing the intake of processed foods, avoiding harmful habits such as smoking and excessive alcohol consumption are all parts of nurturing your temple.

5.3. Training Your Physical Temple

Creating a workout routine that fosters physical strength, flexibility, endurance, balance, and coordination is critical to the transformation. Remember, the aim is not to push the body beyond its limits, but rather, to gently yet distinctly stretch its boundaries, promoting robust physical health.

The workouts should be a balanced mix of Cardiovascular exercises, Strength training, Flexibility exercises, and Balance drills. Each category brings its unique benefits to the temple. Cardiovascular exercises, such as brisk walking, swimming, or cycling help boost heart's health and improve lung capacity. Strength training, with elements such as weight lifting or resistance band workouts, enhance muscle health and bone density. Flexibility exercises, commonly associated with Yoga or Pilates, help keep the muscles supple and joints mobile. Balance drills, often part of martial arts or functional training routines, aid in improving posture and coordination.

Remember to start out slow, though. The sudden or intense activity can potentially lead to injury, defeating the intended purpose of a healthier body. Gradually increase the intensity or duration of each workout session as your body adapts to the current fitness level.

5.4. The Role of Rest and Recovery

As essential it is to engage the body in activity, it is of equal, if not more, importance to allow your body to rest and recover. Punishing workouts with minimal attention paid to rest periods can lead to exhaustion, injury, and burnout.

Recovery should orient around quality sleep and active rest days. Sleep is the prime time when the body heals and refreshes itself. Ensure to get 7-9 hours of sleep daily to facilitate this process optimally. Active rest days are when the body is not subjected to intense workouts but indulged in light activity such as stretching, walking, or meditative practices. These days provide a necessary break to the body while keeping it engaged.

5.5. Immersive Experience with Yoga

Of all the physical workouts in the world, Yoga stands out for its exclusive holistic approach. Originally established by the ancient sages of India, Yoga aims to harmonize the body, mind, and spirit. Body postures, or asanas, breathing techniques, or pranayama, meditative practices, and ethical principles all form part of the Yoga pathway.

Inclusion of yoga into your fitness regimen allows for physical training that is not merely a means to an end, but in itself, a deeply immersive, meditative experience. It enhances strength, flexibility, balance, and also augments internal harmony and tranquility, syncing well with our overarching goal of embodied spirituality.

As you progress on this fitness journey, remember that the goal is not merely to improve your physical strength or endurance but to cultivate a deep, enduring connection with your body, treating it with the love, respect, and diligence it deserves. Reflect often on the progress you have made, not just in expanding physical capacities but in nurturing the body-soul relationship. Treat every moment of nurturing your body as a meditation, as an act of love, and experience the journey of fitness as an enriching, liberating spiritual practice.

Chapter 6. From Samsara to Nirvana: Channeling Mindfulness into Movement

Exploring the path from impermanent worldly existence (Samsara) to the peace of ultimate liberation (Nirvana) in Buddhism, it is enlightening to understand how we can channel the concept of mindfulness into physical movement. It is a sublime journey of harmonizing the body and mind for attaining true wellbeing and inner peace.

6.1. Respecting Your Physical Form

To embrace the Buddha's teachings in our fitness routine, we begin by recognizing and respecting the physical form gifted to us. The human body is said to be a precious and rare opportunity in the cycle of rebirths (Samsara).

It's essential to regard physical fitness as more than a vanity project; it's about keeping the body, an invaluable vehicle for enlightenment, healthy and robust. Each physical exercise can be considered an expression of gratitude towards our bodies - an act of maintaining and honoring it.

The Buddha taught moderation in everything. Too much or too little exercise can harm the body. In line with that, adopting a balanced fitness routine ensures your body gets an optimal workout without being excessively strained.

Tuning into Mindfulness

Mindfulness, or Sati in Pali language, is a significant practice in

Buddhism. It is the aware, equanimous observation of what's happening within us and around us in the present moment. When incorporated into physical activity, it helps synchronize the body and mind and brings harmony to our being.

While performing physical exercises, become mindful of each movement. Observe how your muscles tense and relax, how your body balances, how it reacts to the strain of the exercise, and how your breath flows. Such mindful movements help integrate bodily activities with mind consciousness.

The Contemplation of the Body

One of the main practices in Buddhist meditation is the contemplation of the body (Kāyagatāsati). This practice can be extended to physical activities too. Integrate mindful observation into your movements, contemplating the body as it is.

Understand the impermanence (Anicca), the suffering (Dukkha), and the selflessness (Anatta) of the body. Realize that it is an ever-changing entity, subject to the principle of cause and effect (Karma). Seeing the body in its constituents such as elements (Dhatu) and energy pathways (Nadis) can give a more holistic and in-depth understanding, promoting health and harmony.

Breathing With Awareness

Breath is an essential bridge between the physical and mental world. Mindful breathing techniques (Ānāpānasati) can naturally blend with physical workouts. It provides an anchor for mindfulness and helps inspire a greater synchronization between body and mind.

Whether it's gentle yoga or intense cardio, align it with your breath cycles. Feel the breath as it enters and leaves your nostrils, filling your lungs, and then getting expelled out, carrying away the physical and emotional toxins. Notice the subtle pauses between inhalations and exhalations. This acts as a powerful tool for anchoring you in the present moment and infuses a calm tranquility into your physical exercise.

Nourishing the Body and Mind

Though not directly related to movement, the act of consuming nourishment - both physical and mental - is crucial for a holistic fitness routine.

The Buddha commended mindful eating. Pay mindful attention to the eating process - the colours, the textures, the flavors, the act of chewing, and the feel of swallowing.

Simultaneously, nourish your mind with wholesome thoughts and knowledge. Meditate and read insightful literature. Engage in positive dialogues and mindful social interactions. This practice will allow for developing a vibrant and healthy attitude towards physical fitness and life in general.

6.2. Moving From Samsara to Nirvana

By skillfully integrating mindfulness into your movements, and developing a balanced approach towards physical exercise, you prepare your body and mind for the journey from Samsara to Nirvana.

Channeling mindfulness not only enhances physical strength and flexibility but also improves mental resilience and flexibility. It develops insight, composure, and elevates your fitness experience from just a physical exertion to a profound process of self-discovery and inner tranquility.

Perhaps, one day, amidst a mindful jog or a workout, in the silent alertness and surge of endorphins, you may find yourself immersed in the liberating peace of Nirvana, far from the madding sphere of Samsara.

This journey is indeed one of transformation - a journey where you harness physical strength and endurance, balanced with inner peace and equanimity, moving from the realm of physical Samsara to the sublime peace of Nirvana.

Buddha's Diet: Eating for Mind-Body Wellness

The rhythm of our lives often revolves around what we eat, how we eat, and when we eat. Reflecting back on the wisdom of Buddha, it's evident that food is not merely meant to fill our stomachs, but it plays an essential role in nurturing the mind and spirit. Buddha, through his teachings, proposed a way of life that stands on the grounds of mindfulness, moderation, and compassion, which includes our diet.

The Middle Path: Balance in Eating

According to the Buddha, the path to enlightenment traverses through a balanced life, which he referred to as the 'Middle Path'. This philosophy extends to eating habits as well. The Buddha advocated for neither indulgence nor starvation but a balanced diet to sustain the body.

Buddha said, "To keep the body in good health is a duty, otherwise, we shall not be able to keep our mind strong and clear." A strong body is the residence of a strong mind. Too much food can lead to indulgence and associated bodily ailments, while too little can lead to weakness and inability to focus. There should be balance and mindfulness in consumption.

Mindful Eating: Savor Each Morsel

Within Buddhism, mindfulness forms the basis of all activities, and eating is no exception. To truly understand the concept of mindful eating as per Buddha's teachings, one has to see eating as a conscious act. One should be fully present while consuming food, savoring each morsel, recognizing its nature, its source, its nourishment, and its taste.

Every ingredient in your meal comes from somewhere; it has a life cycle. Recognizing this interdependence signifies being mindful. Enjoying each bite and savoring the taste, the textures, and the aroma allow us to be in the present moment, centring our mind, reducing negative emotions and increasing our appreciation for the world around us.

Nourishment for Mind and Body

Just as a car needs the right fuel to run smoothly, our bodies require the right food to function well. Buddha favored foods that were fresh, natural, and increased clarity of mind and physical stamina.

Fruits, vegetables, whole grains, nuts, seeds and legumes were essentials. Food should provide the right nutrients for the body. But it's not only about the body; the food we eat should assist in mental clarity as well. High-quality natural foods, low in sugars and void of artificial substances, should be preferred over highly processed meals.

Dietary Moderation: Not too Little, Not too Much

The Buddha taught that moderation in food is pivotal to the path towards enlightenment. He recommended monks to consider food as medicine, eating just what the body requires to function optimally. Too little, and the body suffers from deficiencies; too much, and it leads to lethargy and obesity.

Fill two-thirds of your stomach with solid food, leaving one-third for liquids, and the remaining for air, professes a traditional Buddhist rule for moderation. This rule assists in avoiding overeating and promotes better digestion.

Compassionate Eating: Plant-Based Diets

Buddhism strongly emphasizes Ahimsa (non-violence) and compassion for all beings. In this light, Buddha endorsed a plant-based diet. By choosing plant-based foods, one refrains from causing harm to animals, supports sustainability, contributes towards lesser harm to the environment, and aids one's health.

If one chooses to eat meat, it is crucial to ensure that the animal was not slaughtered for one's consumption directly and should be treated humanely during its life.

Walking towards the path of Buddha and practicing his teachings around mindful, balanced, nutritious and compassionate eating not only aids in physical wellness but also fosters mental and spiritual well-being. It's not merely a diet plan, but a lifestyle choice that brings forth harmony with nature, peace with oneself, and attunement with their inner self.

By eating the Buddha's way, the act of consumption becomes an act of mindful meditation, a harmonious dance of the body, mind, and soul. It transfigures our relationship with food, making us realize that eating is not just a mundane task, but an experience of nourishment, gratitude, and joy. This is not only a path towards wellness but also the path towards Enlightenment.

Embrace the Buddha's way of eating and experience a life balanced in body and rich in spirit. The way to spiritual and physical fitness does not remain a far-fetched dream, but a tangible reality within your reach.

Chapter 7. The Art of Meditation: Boosting Physical Health

Meditation is an ancient practice embedded in the heart of various spiritual traditions for centuries. Predominantly known for its lasting impacts on mental health, it is gradually being recognized for its benefits on physical health as well. Inculcating a regular meditation practice and coupling it with physical exercises can indeed bridge the gap between physical well-being and inner tranquility.

Chapter 8. Harnessing the Power of the Mind

The human mind is a powerful tool, capable of influencing physical health to a great extent. A regular, disciplined practice of meditation can help harness this power effectively. It helps quiet the mind, driving away stress and negativity while instilling a sense of peace and positivity. This change in the mental state has visible effects on physical well-being, improving body functions, boosting immunity, and greatly enhancing resilience.

Meditation is simple yet profound, affecting every part of our being. It produces changes in brain activity linked to improved health outcomes. Mindfulness meditation and focused-attention meditation are known to reduce symptoms of physical discomfort, promote better sleep, lower blood pressure, and improve heart health. They are also found to affect the perception of physical pain, thus providing relief.

Chapter 9. The Physiology of Meditation

Meditation impacts several aspects of the body's physiology. It reduces the heart rate and blood pressure, slows down the breathing, and promotes a relaxation response in the body. This relaxed state helps in the recovery and repair of the body's cells and tissues, eventually boosting overall physical health. Moreover, prolonged practice triggers changes at the molecular level, altering gene expression and delaying telomere shortening, factors associated with a reduced aging process and chronic diseases risk.

Chapter 10. Techniques for Physical Wellness

There exist several meditation techniques designed specifically for physical wellness. One such method is Body Scan Meditation, which helps tune into the body and understand its needs better. It directs attention to different parts of the body, noting sensations without judgment. It helps develop mindfulness towards physical discomfort and eases conditions like chronic pain and tension headaches.

Loving-Kindness meditation, often used to cultivate a sense of inner peace and compassion, has shown to have cardiovascular benefits. It reduces the risk of heart disease by promoting emotions like love and compassion, which in turn, trigger the release of the hormone oxytocin, known for its cardioprotective effects.

Another popular technique is Breath-focused meditation. It involves mindful breathing and helps in reducing anxiety, lowering blood pressure, improving lung function, and enhancing cardiovascular health.

Chapter 11. Integrating Meditation into your Fitness Regime

Integrating meditation into your fitness regime necessitates a holistic approach towards health. Start by setting aside dedicated time for meditation. Beginning or ending your workout with meditation can set the correct mindset for the exercise and help your body relax post-workout. It also ensures a deeper connection between the mind and body, enhancing the effectiveness of the workouts.

Always listen to your body and allow it to dictate your fitness schedule. Some days may necessitate more rigorous workouts while on others, a simple stretch routine followed by meditation may suffice. Craft a balanced routine where physical exercises aid strength and endurance building while meditation ensures mental stamina and resilience.

Chapter 12. Results and Benefits: An Overview

Gradually, with consistent practice, the benefits of incorporating meditation into a fitness regime become evident. Reduction in stress levels, improved focus and enhanced recovery times post workouts, are just the first few noticeable changes. In the long run, meditation improves cardiovascular health, reduces chronic pain, promotes better sleep, and boosts the immune function.

Ultimately, a robust practice of meditation coupled with physical exercises leads to a healthy body, an agile mind, and an awakened soul. While physical exercises take care of the visible facets of health and strength, meditation nurtures what lies beneath - our true essence.

In conclusion, achieving physical health through meditation is about growing in awareness, becoming tuned into your body's needs and signals, and establishing a balance between exertion and relaxation. It's about viewing health not merely as the absence of disease but as a profound state of holistic well-being. So, why not twine your fitness routine with this practice of presence and peace?

Chapter 13. Immunity and Inner Peace: Healing from Within

The innate power of the human body to heal itself, boosted by a strong immune system, is an astonishing feature of our intricate biological design. It is a well-established truth that physical health is intertwined with emotional balance and a serenity of spirit. As we venture into the heart of this chapter, we will unveil the profound connection between immunity and inner peace, show how spiritual practices can enhance immune function, and gloriously heal us from within.

13.1. The Connection Between Immunity and Inner Peace

While it might seem counterintuitive initially, there is significant scientific evidence demonstrating a direct correlation between our emotional state and our bodily health. Chronic stress, harbored resentment, and unresolved trauma can wield considerable negative impact on our immune system. Contrarily, inner peace – the profound state of tranquility and harmony within oneself – boosts resilience, enhancing our body's natural ability to resist infections and disease.

Emerging research suggests that stress reduction techniques, meditation, and various spiritual practices augment immune function, largely mediated through stress hormone modulation and anti-inflammatory pathways. These practices have been associated with decreased cortisol levels, improved production of white blood cells, and a boost in the bodies' natural killer cells, all imperative for a healthy immune system. Our body and mind are not disparate, but function in harmony, interconnected in ways often too profound for the eye to see.

13.2. Spiritual Practices to Boost Immunity

Boosting immunity is not merely a matter of popping multivitamin pills or adhering to strict dietary regimes. Inner peace, attained via spiritual practices, holds the key to bolstering our defenses. Here, we will explore some practices that can pave the way towards enhanced immune health.

1. **Mindfulness Meditation:** Practiced since ancient times, mindfulness meditation sharpens our focus on the present moment, eschewing rumination over the past or anxiety for the future. Consciously focusing on our breath or an chosen object can work wonders in calming our frenzied minds. Far from being esoteric, the rewards of mindfulness have been backed by rigorous scientific studies displaying enhanced immune response, straightening the marvelous mind-body link.

2. **Yoga:** This ancient, multi-dimensional practice includes postures (asanas), controlled breathing (pranayama), and meditation, harmoniously blending physical exertion and mental tranquility. Regular practice of yoga can increase endurance, flexibility, and balance, alongside stress reduction and immune enhancement.

3. **Tai Chi:** Known as 'meditation in motion', Tai Chi is a non-competitive, self-paced system of gentle physical exercises and stretching. Constant focus on body movements can help the practitioner to stay in the present moment, liberating the mind from scattered thoughts. Studies suggest promising effects of Tai Chi on immune function, particularly in older adults.

13.3. Healing Mind, Body, and Spirit with Nutrition

While physical workouts and meditative practices greatly contribute to our well-being, it's crucial not to ignore the role of nutrition. Adopting a balanced diet provides the necessary nutrients required to maintain a healthy immune system. Fresh fruits and vegetables, whole grains, lean proteins, and healthy fats should be balanced in our daily meals. Consuming food should not be viewed as fuelling our bodies alone, but as a holistic practice where we nourish our body as well as our spirit.

A holistic approach to immunity involves conscientious adherence to a nutritious diet, amalgamated with spiritual practices focused on evoking inner peace. The journey towards health is not a destination, but an ongoing path where wellness presents as joyous living – where existential wellbeing synergizes with physical vigor, creating a symphony of harmonized existence.

13.4. Embrace the Multi-dimensional Approach

Embarking on a journey towards improved immunity, finding a path to inner peace, and healing from within is a multi-faced venture. It involves a deep commitment to personal growth, disciplined lifestyle choices, and a genuine effort to connect deeply with oneself. This chapter has attempted to guide you on this journey, highlighting the deep-seated interdependence of immunity and inner peace, and showing how spiritual practices can contribute to physical well-being. Let this understanding invigorate your path towards holistic health, influencing every choice you make, from the food you consume, the activities you engage in, and the thoughts you entertain.

In the end, it's important to remember that attaining inner peace or regularizing immunity does not happen overnight. It's a beautiful journey of self-realization and growth. As you take each step on this path, remember that every effort counts towards achieving harmony between your body, mind, and spirit - this is the essence of true wellness and the potent secret of healing from within.

"The secret of health for both mind and body is not to mourn for the past, nor to worry about the future, but to live the present moment wisely and earnestly." - Gautama Buddha

Chapter 14. Mind and Matter: The Synergy of Mental and Physical Stamina

Our journey commences from an area where our mental and physical realms interweave, manifesting as stamina. The synergy of mental and physical stamina is a potent combination that facilitates not only better body strength but also mental resilience. Delving deep into this connection, we'll explore how we can strengthen these ties and foster a mutually nourishing relationship between our mental and physical aspects.

14.1. Unveiling the Connection

It's often easy to segregate our mind from our physical being, considering them to exist in entirely separate realms. Yet, they're intrinsically woven in a loop of constant influence. The mind influences the body, the body influences the mind. Understanding this subtle relationship is the cornerstone of achieving holistic health.

Psychoneuroimmunology, an evolved field of study, inspects these interrelationships closely. This science outlines the pathways and connections between our nervous system, immune system, and our mental state. Research in this science has revealed evidence pointing towards the significant impact our mindset holds over our physical health, and vice versa.

Studies have shown that continuous states of mental stress have a tangible impact on our physical health. Chronic stress contributes to higher rates of heart diseases, worsens respiratory ailments, and can trigger or exacerbate gastrointestinal problems. So, if the mind can inflict physical ailment, it holds true that a healthier mental state can result in better physical health and stamina.

14.2. Boosting Physical Stamina: The Outer Work

Physical stamina is built through intentional, rigorous physical training and a balanced diet. This is the outer work required, which gives your body the strength and stamina to go farther and perform for extended periods.

Integrating exercise into daily routines is step one towards a stronger physique. Exploring different forms of exercise such as cardiovascular workouts, resistance training, yoga, and mindful practices like Tai Chi can add variety and enhance the efficacy of fitness routines.

Recollect the wisdom of Buddha, "To keep the body in good health is a duty." Consistent, targeted workouts promote muscle development, improve cardiovascular health, and enhance the body's overall endurance levels.

A balanced diet cannot be overlooked in the pursuit of better physical stamina. It's necessary to intake a variety of nutrients that help the body recover and build stamina. Hydrate adequately, incorporate protein-rich foods that facilitate muscle repair and growth, and complex carbohydrates for sustained energy levels.

14.3. Inner Work: Boosting Mental Stamina

As you work on refining your physical stamina, it's equally crucial to focus on mental stamina. Your mind ought to have the resilience to endure, overcome obstacles, and carry on despite challenges. Sanskrit scriptures describe it as "Dhairyam," the courage or mental strength achieved through the practice of discipline and patience.

Mental stamina can be fostered through consistent mindfulness practices – the heart of Buddha's teachings. Mindfulness not only reduces stress and anxiety but also trains your mind to focus and develop mental fortitude.

Consider incorporating meditation in your fitness routine. Start off with brief periods, gradually increasing time as you grow comfortable. Mindfulness isn't only for a set meditation time; try to carry this awareness throughout your day, being mindful of your actions, thoughts, and feelings.

Another effective mental practice is visualization. Visualize yourself as strong and resilient. Think about how you can move with grace and strength. Picture yourself meeting your fitness goals. This understanding creates a drive, an internal pull enabling you to push through barriers, thereby enhancing your stamina.

14.4. Synergy of Stamina: Where Mind and Body Meet

When you start working on enhancing both physical and mental stamina, you'll notice an increasing synergy between your mind and body. Your body will respond better when your mind is focused, and your mind will have the ability to push the body beyond the presumed limitations.

The Buddha has advised, "It is better to conquer yourself than to win a thousand battles." With regular practice, you'll find yourself achieving targets you deemed unlikely before. The robust stamina you developed from your physical workouts will intertwine with mental stability obtained from mindfulness practices, promoting an evolved self that possesses a fortified mind-body connection.

The holistic exercise is indeed a harmonious dance between the physical and the spiritual - one where sweat meets tranquility, and where strength greets peace.

Wrapping up this exploration of the synergy of mental and physical stamina, we hope you've gained insights and are inspired to blend these practices in your life. Establishing a dynamic balance between physical fitness and mental fortitude is not just a path to a healthier body, but it's also a journey towards an invigorated and serene mind. This is where the purpose of our endeavor lies - in the beautiful balance and unison of the physical and spiritual, creating a realm of well-being that's richly rewarding.

Chapter 15. Ethical Living for Good Health: The Five Precepts of Buddha

Buddhism is not only a religion or a philosophy, but a significant spiritual journey towards achieving enlightenment. The journey starts from within, transforming every aspect of life, including our physical health. Within its tenants, Buddhism elucidates a unique path of maintaining and enhancing a robust physique, mental positivity, and overall well-being.

At the core of Buddhism lie the 'Five Precepts.' Being an essential part of the Buddha's teachings, these precepts act as the guiding principles for an ethical life, directly impacting one's physical health. They are not strict commandments to bind the practitioners. Rather, they are a set of voluntarily acknowledged moral guidelines that help foster a harmonious living that, in turn, brings good health.

Let's delve into these five precepts and understand how they contribute towards healthful living.

15.1. The First Precept: Abstaining from Taking Life

The first precept emphasizes non-violence and reverence for life. It signifies abstaining from causing harm to any living creature, promoting peace in our surroundings and within ourselves. By practicing this precept, we develop compassion for ourselves and every life form around us.

According to current research, compassion can lead to lower stress levels, healthier hearts, and a stronger immune system. Practicing non-violence and compassion can help form healthy habits such as choosing a balanced diet that emphasizes plant-based options. It can also improve mental health by mitigating hostile impulses and promoting a general sense of peace.

15.2. The Second Precept: Abstaining from Taking What Is Not Given

This precept is about respect for others' rights and property. It extends to developing ethical behavior in our dealing with the materialistic world, establishing honesty, trust, and integrity. Consequently, it contributes to developing emotional health by reducing the stress and guilt associated with deceptive behaviors.

Practicing this precept could lead to less societal stress, fostering a sense of peace in our daily life. Accepting and respecting other people's possessions (both material and immaterial) eliminates the negative feelings such as jealousy, greed, and resentment, promoting overall emotional health and stability.

15.3. The Third Precept: Abstaining from Sexual Misconduct

This precept guides the formulation of ethical, responsible, and loving relationships. It emphasizes mutual respect in relationships, fostering empathy and harmony. By discouraging unhealthy sexual behaviors, it further contributes to physical health by minimizing sexually transmitted diseases and potential mental health issues emerging from unhealthy relationships.

The practice of this precept leads to mindful actions in relationships, causing less harm to oneself and others. It promotes understanding, therefore reducing relationship stress and related mental health issues.

15.4. The Fourth Precept: Abstaining from False Speech

The fourth precept pertains to practicing truthfulness and abstaining from deceitful speech. This involves not only avoiding lies but also abstaining from slanderous talk, harsh words, and frivolous chatter. This moral decorum stipulates honesty, which aids in maintaining a clear conscience, leading to lesser mental stress and better mental health.

Practicing mindful speech can reduce potential misunderstandings, man-made conflicts, and increase trust amongst individuals. Clear, honest, and mindful communication can significantly enhance emotional health and foster positive relationships.

15.5. The Fifth Precept: Abstaining from Intoxicants

The fifth precept prohibits the consumption of intoxicants that lead to heedlessness. Intoxicants obscure the clarity of mind, making it difficult to comply with other precepts. By adhering to this precept, we maintain physical health by avoiding the harmful effects of alcohol, drugs, and other intoxicants on the body.

In addition to physical health, this precept sustains mental health and emotional well-being by ensuring clarity of mind and emotional stability, improving overall quality of life.

In conclusion, the Five Precepts of Buddha form a guide to ethical living that promotes holistic well-being. Adherence to these precepts contributes to molding a life characterized by peace, compassion, and harmony, resulting in better physical health, mental health, and overall well-being. By imparting a simple yet profound lifestyle guideline, Buddha's teachings enable us to lead an ethical life that directly contributes to good health.

Chapter 16. Keeping the Balance: Daily Practices for Holistic Well-being

Daily practices for holistic well-being require a careful balance between physical health, mental strength, and spiritual tranquility. In this multifaceted journey, will be discovered the synergy between fitness and mindfulness, integrating the two into a personalized daily routine that fosters both bodily wellness and inner peace. This path begins with the basics: understanding balance and approaching the three pillars of holistic well-being.

16.1. Understanding Balance

One must first apprehend the importance of balance. Balance isn't about uniformity or homogenization. Rather, it is an understanding of our own unique needs and capacities, and harmonizing our mind, body, and spirit accordingly. A healthy body is useless without a peaceful mind, and a peaceful mind gets weaker without a healthy body. Spiritual practices are foundational to achieving this balance, setting aligned energy and intentions for personal health and calmness.

16.2. The Three Pillars of Holistic Well-being

Holistic well-being rests on three fundamental pillars: body, mind, and spirit. None of these pillars can stand alone, and so the key to achieving holistic health is to ensure that all three are equally supported and developed.

1. **Body**: Maintaining physical health and strength through regular exercise, a balanced diet, and a proper sleep schedule. This may involve various forms of physical activity, from leisurely walking to more rigorous routines like yoga or martial arts.

2. **Mind**: Boosting mental health by managing stress, engaging in regular self-reflection, and nurturing a positive, growth-oriented mindset. Mind strength also involves self-expression, creativity, learning, and engagement in activities that bring joy and contentment.

3. **Spirit**: Cultivating spirituality through practices that connect you to a larger purpose or higher power. This could take the form of meditation, mindfulness, prayer, or activities that bring a sense of peace and perspective.

16.3. Integrating Mindful Fitness into Daily Routine

The integration of physical exercise with mindfulness can act as a powerful catalyst for holistic wellness. Regular physical activity promotes strength, agility, and cardiovascular health, while mindfulness exercises help mitigate stress, improve mental clarity, and foster inner peace. Some practices that fuse both include:

- **Mindful Morning Exercise**: Kickstart your day with a gentle physical activity, like a morning walk or sun salutation yoga sequence. Emphasize mind-body awareness, feeling each movement and breath as you engage your body.

- **Midday Stretch and Calm**: A simple set of stretches coupled with a short mindfulness or meditation exercise can be an excellent break in the lunch hour, promoting calmness, reducing stress, and boosting your afternoon productivity.

- **Evening Unwind**: Normalizing a routine to unwind before sleep that includes light yoga postures and a mindfulness practice can aid in better sleep and relaxation.

16.4. The Role of Nutrition in Holistic Well-being

A balanced diet is a vital element of physical health and has significant influence over mental and spiritual well-being too. Consuming nutritious, wholesome food fuels the body adequately, supports cognition, and invites a sense of divine appreciation for the food you consume.

A holistic approach to diet includes the following:

1. **Conscious Eating**: Be fully aware of what you eat, where it comes from, and how it's prepared. This mindfulness can enhance your relationship with food and lead to healthier eating habits.

2. **Variety and Balance**: Include diverse food items from all food groups in right proportions to ensure a rich supply of necessary nutrients.

3. **Organic and Natural Foods**: Aim to consume more organic, real food, which are free from harmful pesticides and are often more nutrient-dense.

16.5. Stress Management and Mental Strength

While physical exercise and balanced nutrition are essential for bodily health, mental strength is equally important in achieving holistic well-being. Stress management, in particular, is critical to mental health and can be gained through the below practices:

- **Mindfulness**: Taking out time each day to focus on being present and fully engaged in the current moment helps in reducing stress and anxiety.

- **Journaling**: Writing down thoughts and feelings can be an effective outlet for stress and serves to improve self-understanding.

- **Practicing gratitude**: Regularly acknowledging and appreciating the positive elements in life can promote a optimistic mindset and counteract the effects of stress.

16.6. Nurturing Spirit through Meditation and Mindfulness

The spirit is invigorated through connection—to oneself, to others, to nature, and to the universe. This connection is nurtured through practices like meditation and mindfulness, that guide towards a deeper understanding of oneself and one's place in the world. Daily meditative practices can include:

- **Silent Meditation**: Reserved time in solitude, focusing on breath or a chosen word or phrase helps in building spiritual strength.

- **Mindful Walks**: Walking mindfully, acknowledging each step and the beauty around helps nurture gratitude, presence, and connection.

- **Loving-kindness Meditation**: This method involves focusing on developing feelings of compassion, love, and kindness towards oneself and others.

Incorporating these different elements into daily life may take time and continuous effort, requiring learning and unlearning. However, the journey towards holistic well-being is a personal and transformative one, and every small step in this direction is an achievement in itself. The equilibrium of the body, mind, and spirit is steadily attained not through drastic change, but through a series of small adjustments, eventually guiding towards a sustained state of harmony and health. All of these practices collectively contribute to a holistic lifestyle that fuels not just physical health, but also a calm and focused mind.